FITMEALS

EAT HEALTHY & STAY FIT

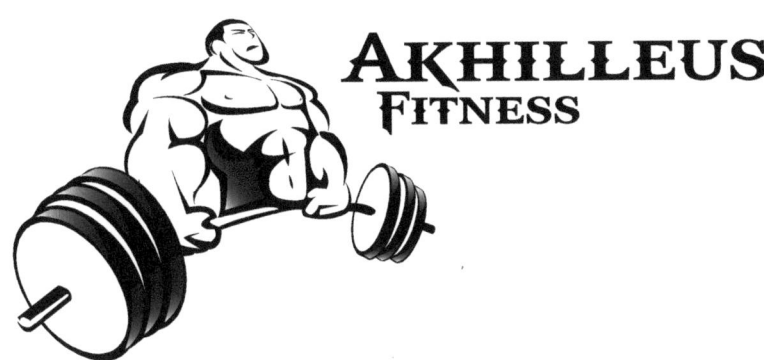

Cover & Book design
© 2014 by Akhilleus Fitness, *Sébastien Leria, Los Angeles, CA*

Editing
Golbarg Hiekali

Cover Photo Credit
Rex Vincent Photography

DEDICATION

As a fitness professional attempting for the first time to convey a message to the masses, I dedicate this book to everyone who has believed in me and my quest to help average people realize their full potential. For every food lover wanting to live and maintain a healthy lifestyle — this is for you.

I would like to thank my family in France, Martinique, and my friends worldwide. Thank you to Goli, for being my support at all times and helping me make this happen. With you at my side, I persevered. Thanks to my Canadian friend Sara, who has helped bring forth ideas and motivation for this book during our casual conversations. There is nothing more exciting than sharing this success with you too. A special thank you to my Greek sister Sotiria, who nicknamed me "Akhilleus," and ignited the spark of my love for fitness and its lifestyle.

And finally, thank you to you, the reader. Your confidence encourages me to continue to help. I am always aiming to produce high-end content with the hope that my words will illustrate my passion. I truly wish to touch your heart and stimulate your own passions towards positive change, and for me to be a continuing inspiration for you to reach your fitness goals. To succeed, the recipe is simple: Take a bit of your willpower, add the support of your loved ones, and have faith. Nothing will remain out of reach. Believe in yourself, because there is nothing you can't do.

Warmly,

Sébastien Leria

TABLE OF CONTENTS

Whoever walks in integrity walks securely,
but whoever takes crooked paths will be
found out.

- Proverbs 10:9

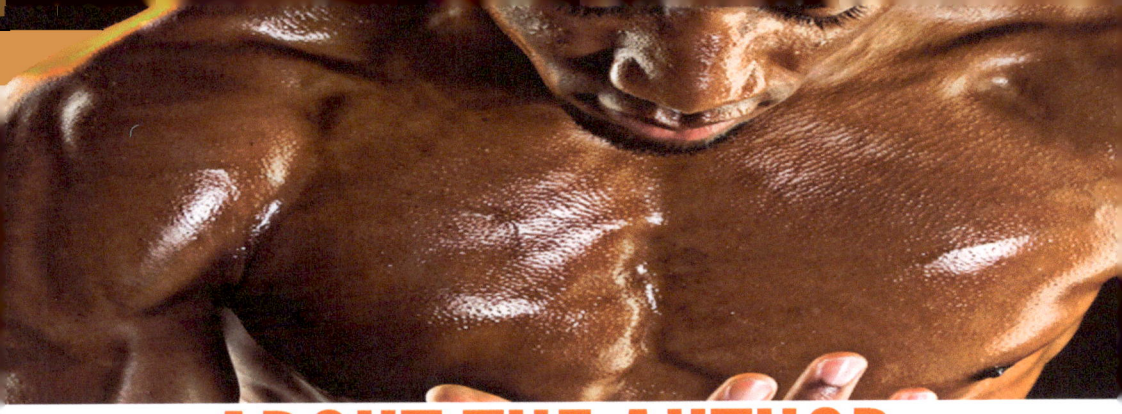

ABOUT THE AUTHOR

Founder of Akhilleus Fitness, ProPTA director of France, fitness model and personal trainer, Sébastien "Akhilleus" Leria is an international athlete and trusted expert on health and fitness. Leria began his career in Europe as a break-dancer and martial artist. His fascination with the improvement of the human form developed as he sculpted his naturally thin body into that of a fitness model.

Out of his passion for helping people achieve health, wellness, and a love of their bodies, Leria created Akhilleus Fitness. Through his company, Leria provides training, consulting and personal guidance to empower people to reach their fitness and health lifestyle goals.Leria's diverse background and training in Body Building, Martial Arts, and Dance has led him to create innovative conditioning techniques that deliver incredible results to clients at all fitness levels and stages. He is certified by the IFBB Professional League in Personal Training and Nutrition.

Akhilleus Fitness consultations are available in-person in Los Angeles, California, Paris, and France or via Skype/Google and e-mail for international clientele. Sébastien Leria's love of health and wellness is positively contagious, and he is honored to support clients on their mission to achieve a body they love and that serves them well, for a lifetime.

DISCLAIMER & MEDICAL CLEARANCE

The material (including without limitation, advice and recommendation) within this guide is provided solely as general educational and informational purposes. Use of this book of recipes, and information contained herein is at the sole choice and risk of the reader. Always consult your physician or healthcare provider before beginning any nutrition program.

If you choose to use this information without the prior consent of your physician, you are agreeing to accept full responsibility for your decisions and are agreeing to hold harmless Akhilleus Fitness, its agents, employees, contractors and any affiliated companies from any liability with respect to injury or illness to you or your property arising out of or connected with your use of the information contained within this book, or our website.

You agree to defend, indemnify, and hold harmless Akhilleus Fitness and other affiliated companies, and their employees, contractors, officers, and directors from all liabilities, claims, and expenses, including attorney's fees, that arise from your use or misuse of your exercise and nutrition programs or other information made available on the website.

THE SECRET BEHIND MY TRANSFORMATION

MAKE YOUR BODY AN ALLY, INSTEAD OF AN OPPONENT

S ome people believe that they know everything about nutrition. Stop right there. This is false. This is what I like to call the "Know-It-All Syndrome." What many people might think is good nutritional advice, may in reality be inaccurate information provided to you by the food industry, eager to sell products.

Let me be clear and straight with you. When a nutritionist tells you to eat or follow a specific regimen, while their own appearance is that of an out of shape and weak individual, this should raise some major red flags. I wouldn't feel completely safe to rely on this person for effective advice on nutrition. Similarly, an obese personal trainer who gives diet tips is not someone who reflects the fitness look they are supposedly advocating. Don't miss the signs. Proponents of healthy nutrition and fitness should directly reflect what they preach.

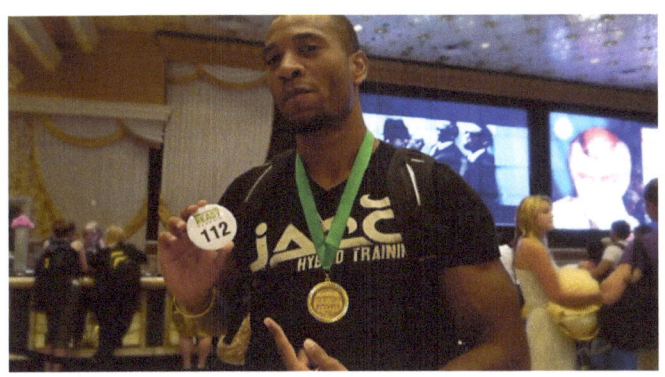

In about two years of dedication.
I went from skeleton and sick looking to self-made Fitness Model & Men's Physique Competitor.

MAKE YOUR BODY AN ALLY, INSTEAD OF AN OPPONENT

These inconsistent systems do not even take into account the importance of the combination of food intake as well as exercise. If a nutritionist is solely focused on preparing a meal plan geared towards your optimal health, he may not be teaching you ways in which you should be incorporating physical training into your daily life in order to reach your desired fitness goals. In addition, most personal trainers are only equipped to provide you with ways in which you can improve your physicality through exercise and may fall short on suggesting healthy foods to eat. Meanwhile, their clients may be eating poorly and not seeing any weight improvements.

Additionally, there are some doctors who generally advise their patients to incorporate some foods into their diet, without taking the time to evaluate what specific foods their patients' bodies will particularly benefit from. I am certainly not stating that all doctors conform to this practice, though I have personally come across a few in my lifetime who have proven to give some questionable advice on food consumption.

As a teenager in high school, I was mocked and bullied by my classmates because of my weight and body type. As an ectomorph, gaining weight has always been extremely difficult for me, whether it be gaining fat tissue or lean mass. When I consulted my doctor regarding this issue, he simply suggested that all I needed to do to gain weight was to "eat a lot of red meat, chicken, and fish" in order to build mass and break down my lean abdominal wall. Of course, it wasn't that simple.

MAKE YOUR BODY AN ALLY, INSTEAD OF AN OPPONENT

After hearing this advice, I truly ate as much meat, chicken, and fish as I could, but the advice was not completely valuable without further explanation and understanding. I did not understand the meaning of "abdominal wall." Today I know that it meant building an extra layer of fat tissue over my muscle, or what we call "bulking". At that time, completely unaware of the process related to nutrition and fitness, I feared that breaking down my lean abdominal wall meant allowing myself to become fat which was a prospect I quickly rejected since it would mean losing the only muscle I was proud to have. Without the proper knowledge and advice, I was eager to maintain my lean abdominals and even challenged myself to incorporate more sit-ups into my daily routine. As a result, instead of building muscle, I found myself bloated, over exhausted and unsatisfied. My doctor's advice lacked sufficient information. Still, I was determined to turn the mockery I was faced with, into respect and admiration; but I was misinformed on how to achieve my goal. I was burning all my calories and was training negatively. I did not build muscle, but only destroyed what my body already had. This experience taught me that few doctors are actually trained to give specific nutrition advice. This is backed up by an article written by the New York Times called, "Teaching Doctors about Nutrition and Diet" published in 2010. Doctors study the general medical curriculum, but nutrition, food, and exercise are just one topic of the large spectrum. Most doctors are not aware or educated in the specific digestion and biochemical reactions that are associated to each specific body type. In my case, my doctor should have focused on giving me a more detailed and informative explanation of what I should do in order to gain more weight. It would have been helpful if he explained the process the body takes and how digestion plays a role as well. An advantageous discovery would have been receiving information on the benefits of supplying my body with meat. He didn't provide me with reasons why I should add more to my diet. Suggesting that I balance my meals with carbohydrates and proteins would have given me concrete knowledge that I could take with me in the future while living my day-to-day life.

MAKE YOUR BODY AN ALLY, INSTEAD OF AN OPPONENT

He should have informed me that balancing my meals with carbs would allow me to build muscle without burning through my lean body mass after an intense workout. Also, it would have been beneficial for him to let me know that eating more protein could help me to build more muscle and create a stronger frame, in spite of my difficult-to-overcome ectomorph genes Now, the Bro-Science; your worst and strongest enemy. Has anyone ever come up to you and told you, "Hey bro! If you wanna get big, start eating all the food you see in front of you. You will get buff in a blink of an eye." Well, it has definitely happened to me. I was desperate for fast results and wasn't getting the expected outcome after following my doctor's advice. I seriously considered eating all of the food I could possibly eat and thought that my body would have no choice but to grow at least some muscles with all that food right? WRONG!! It was the worst decision I had ever made, not to mention a very unhealthy one. Day after day I continued to eat processed foods filled with preservatives. Junk food, fast food, I ate it all. This led to food intoxication, which results from the consumption of toxins or poisons that are produced in food through bacterial growth. Because of this, I consulted three specialists and even had to undergo an ultrasound to ensure that no organs were inflamed and that the pain in my abdomen was not due to kidney stones or any condition other than food intoxication. Did I gain weight? Did I obtain lean mass? Yes, I did. But the cost of the pain and unhealthy damage I caused to my body was not worth it, nor appealing anymore. I went too far in the process of wanting to gain weight and I learned from it. When I mention "junk food", I am referring to foods that are relatively high in caloric content, but low in nutritional value. They are often high in salt, sugar, white flour and saturated fat. These foods are usually processed and prepackaged which makes it easy to prepare and consume, but in no way exerts the meaning of the word "healthy." It is not enough to just eat well sometimes, and eat junk and unhealthy meals at other times. Fitness and nutrition go hand in hand.

MAKE YOUR BODY AN ALLY, INSTEAD OF AN OPPONENT

Consistency is key. First you need to become aware of what your body specifically needs in order to maintain a healthy anatomical system. Then you can make it a point to eat precisely what your body needs in order to stimulate hypertrophy and cellular regeneration. Even for me, as a formerly "skinny" guy, poor quality food will leave me extremely ill.

Furthermore, the effects on an obese person eating the same junk I ate would be even more detrimental considering their vital organs may already be filled with fat. This can result in obesity, diabetes, high cholesterol, blood pressure, and can contribute to heart disease. Think twice before drinking a Big Gulp next time. All of this made me recognize that my lack of knowledge on the topic of nutrition was the main issue. I began to study what the best foods are for different body types, and it's something I continue to learn about each day. I was able to figure out what works and what doesn't. I experimented on myself and conducted research in order to learn more about the effects of different types of food on the body.

Now I have finally reached the look of a Fitness Model and have proudly competed in Men's Physique competitions. All of the mockery I was faced with inadvertently helped me become a better person that constantly strives to improve himself. Today, I clearly understand that even optimal nutrition plus impeccable training methods cannot achieve superior results, if put into action only independently; They truly work hand in hand.

MAKE YOUR BODY AN ALLY, INSTEAD OF AN OPPONENT

Below is a picture of me before and after my life changing experience. I think you will be able to notice the difference... I didn't know much about nutrition and this also applies to most North American doctors. Many of them have never studied nutrition. In fact, most are not specialized in that sector. If you do your homework and research this topic, you will be amazed and possibly shocked at how little doctors actually know about nutrition. Don't be fooled by Dr. OZ's tips, the South Beach Diet, the Dukan or even the Parisian Diet. Open your eyes, wake up, and begin to learn. The only diet that works is the "DO-IT-YOURSELF DIET."

I would like to take you on this road filled with unlimited resources of knowledge to help you achieve your personal goals, with simple baby steps. There is no rush and no pressure. Let's start your new food adventure!

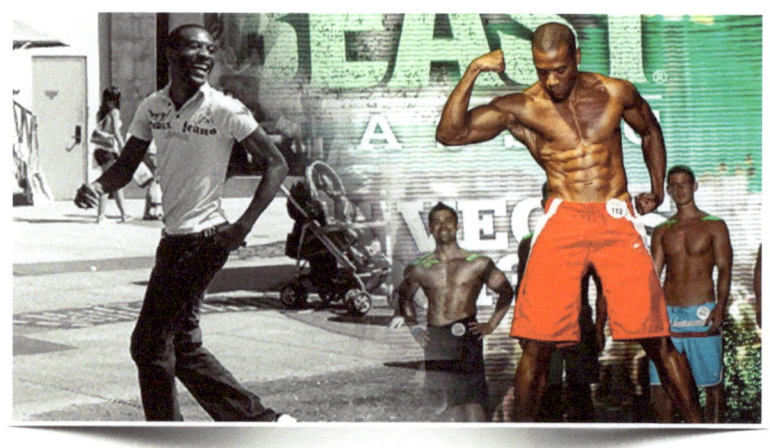

MAKE YOUR BODY AN ALLY, INSTEAD OF AN OPPONENT

I didn't know much about nutrition and this also applies to most North American doctors. Many of them have never studied nutrition. In fact, most are not specialized in that sector. If you do your homework and research this topic, you will be amazed and possibly shocked at how little doctors actually know about nutrition. Don't be fooled by Dr. OZ's tips, the South Beach Diet, the Dukan or even the Parisian Diet. Open your eyes, wake up, and begin to learn. The only diet that works is the "DO-IT-YOURSELF DIET."

I would like to take you on this road filled with unlimited resources of knowledge to help you achieve your personal goals, with simple baby steps. There is no rush and no pressure. Let's start your new food adventure!

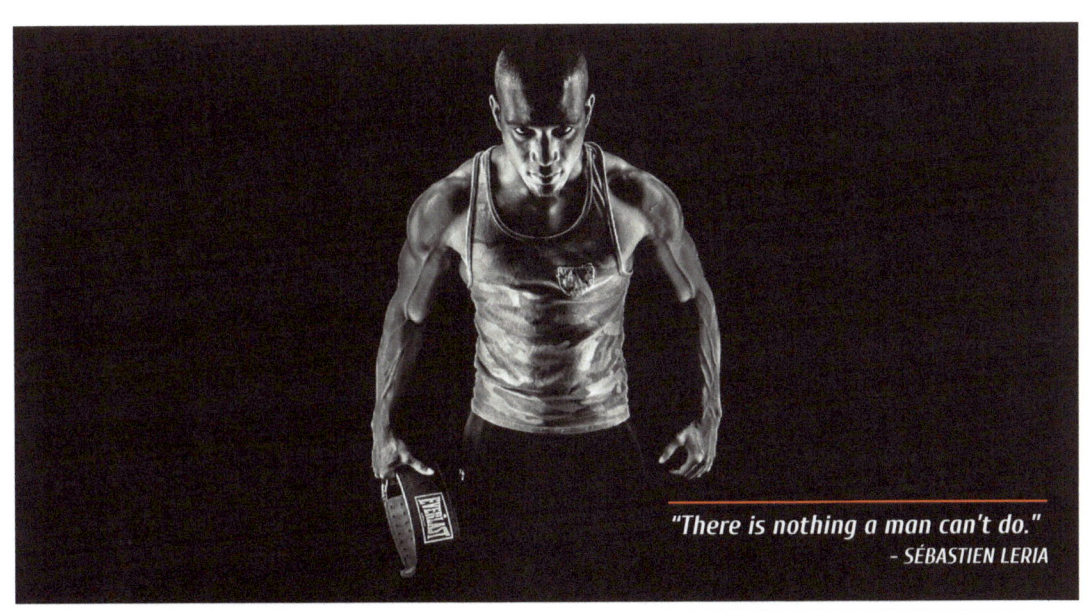

"There is nothing a man can't do."
- SÉBASTIEN LERIA

Therefore, having put away falsehood, let each one of you speak the truth with his neighbor, for we are members one of another.

- *Ephesians 4:25*

THIS IS NOT A DIET

This book is quite simple to use. I have written it in such a way that allows you to reproduce all the different recipes provided. It will also give you the tools and ability to create new recipes without much effort. I have provided you with information that can be applied to you in various ways, depending on your fitness needs and goals.

The recipes I have included are the same ones I used for myself during my fitness journey. After experimenting with different ingredients and dietary combinations, I have finally put together some fitness-friendly and appetizing dishes that are both delicious and healthy. I am excited and proud to share with you the results of my extensive "Gourmet Research."

I always strive for accuracy and attention to detail, which is why I have created this book in an easy-to-read and concise manner - providing you with correct and streamlined information. To that end, I invite you read overly the "Fitness Tips" section of this book. You will find in-depth explanations that justify the need to eat balanced meals. The key is to cover the full spectrum of a nutritional plan, which includes: Proteins/Carbs/Fats.

My intention is not to ask the readers of this book to start a "diet". My true desire is to help you to understand the best manner in which to organize a meal with the inclusion of all the necessary macronutrients. I intend to share everything I have learned with the specific goal of equipping readers with the knowledge to effectively review their eating habits and appropriately monitor their food intake.

While our bodies may lead us to different destinations, control over our food will make the fitness journey an effective and rewarding process to take.

THIS IS NOT A DIET

As a certified nutrition technician, I can't stress enough the simple fact that Proteins, Carbohydrates, Fats and Water are mandatory in any meal plan to maintain an optimal health level. It is required that you include all of these elements in your meal. In the next section, you will find that I have compiled some useful data regarding this area.

The following chapters will supply you with an optimized and compelling outlook that you have undoubtedly come to expect with the purchase of this book. I take this opportunity to congratulate you in advance. The decision you made to learn from this nutrition guide will truly impact your life if you read it carefully and the way it is designed to support you.

I am thankful for your faith in me and hope to help you in the best way that I can. Now venture forth into the following mouth-watering chapters. Eat good food and spread the word that eating healthy is fun, tasty and a real life pleasure like nothing else.

INTRODUCTION

Who, What, and Why?

Proper nutrition is important to everyone because it allows the body to absorb the required nutrients to stay healthy, grow and work efficiently. The quality of your food intake will have a direct effect on your metabolic activity. Nutrition is mostly seen as the combination of our most important basic necessities, such as food and water. As most of us probably know, foods are made up of six classes of nutrients. Good nutrition means getting enough macronutrients. Macronutrients contain Proteins, Carbohydrates, and Fats. Micronutrients include water, vitamins and minerals. Each nutrient has a unique and vital role to play in efficient bodily functions. For a better quality of life, it's recommended to incorporate a regular Weight Training activity to promote hormones and cell regeneration within your organism. Losing weight and keeping it off is more complicated than eating a specific

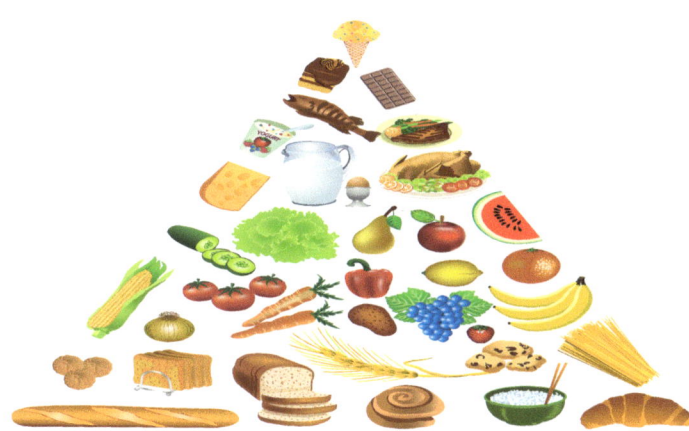

Your muscles need energy to work, so the more muscle mass you have, the more calories you burn over the course of the day.

It works like this for every pound of muscle you gain. You will burn 35-50 more calories a day. Now that is a reason to stimulate a strength-training addition in your routine. Let's breakdown the six classes mentioned above — it will provide a complimentary foundation of the need to eat enough to replenish and feed that precious lean body mass.

amount of calories and lowering it to produce weight loss. While following a nutritional plan, strength training is vital or else you risk losing more lean muscle mass rather than losing adipose tissue, (fat cells) which are very important to keep your metabolism going.

MACRONUTRIENTS

CARBOHYDRATES

There are two types of carbohydrates: simple and complex. The simple carbohydrates include refined sugars and sugars that occur naturally (e.g. white sugar, sugar found in fruits.) The complex carbohydrate can be found in foods such as pasta and vegetables. They give you energy and are very valuable to your body. The main function of a Carbohydrate is to supply the body with energy while it digests food.

Carbohydrates are broken down into a substance that the bloodstream uses to feed your muscles, organs and brain. They contribute to the formation of cellular constituents. Your daily Carbohydrate intake should be around 60 percent of your food intake.

FATS

While most of us tend to avoid fat, it's very important to recognize the role that it plays from a nutritional point of view. Fats insulate your whole body and protect nerve pathways, as well as your organs. Fat is a mandatory part of proper nutrition as it allows fat-soluble vitamins to spread throughout your body. You must ingest fat wisely and be careful of the amount or type of fat you include in your diet. Fats are classified under the following types: saturated and unsaturated.

Saturated fat can be found in solid form at room temperature and can be harmful for your arteries as they cause blockages. On the other hand, unsaturated fats are less likely to pack together and cause blockage of the arteries, but it can still occur in certain cases. The best source of unsaturated fat can be found in olives, peanuts and walnuts. It is generally recommended to get an average of 20 - 30 percent of your daily calories from fat. It goes without saying that it's more beneficial to select unsaturated fats to include in your diet to maintain a healthy lifestyle

MACRONUTRIENTS

PROTEINS

Protein helps to build muscle; the body's tissue growth reinforces the immune system and promotes healing. Proteins supply amino acids and contribute to the formation of enzymes as well as hormones. They are the largest group of nutrients present in the human body. They also aid in the development of antibodies. They play an important role in our metabolic response. It is recommended that you get an average of 20% to 30% protein from your daily calories.

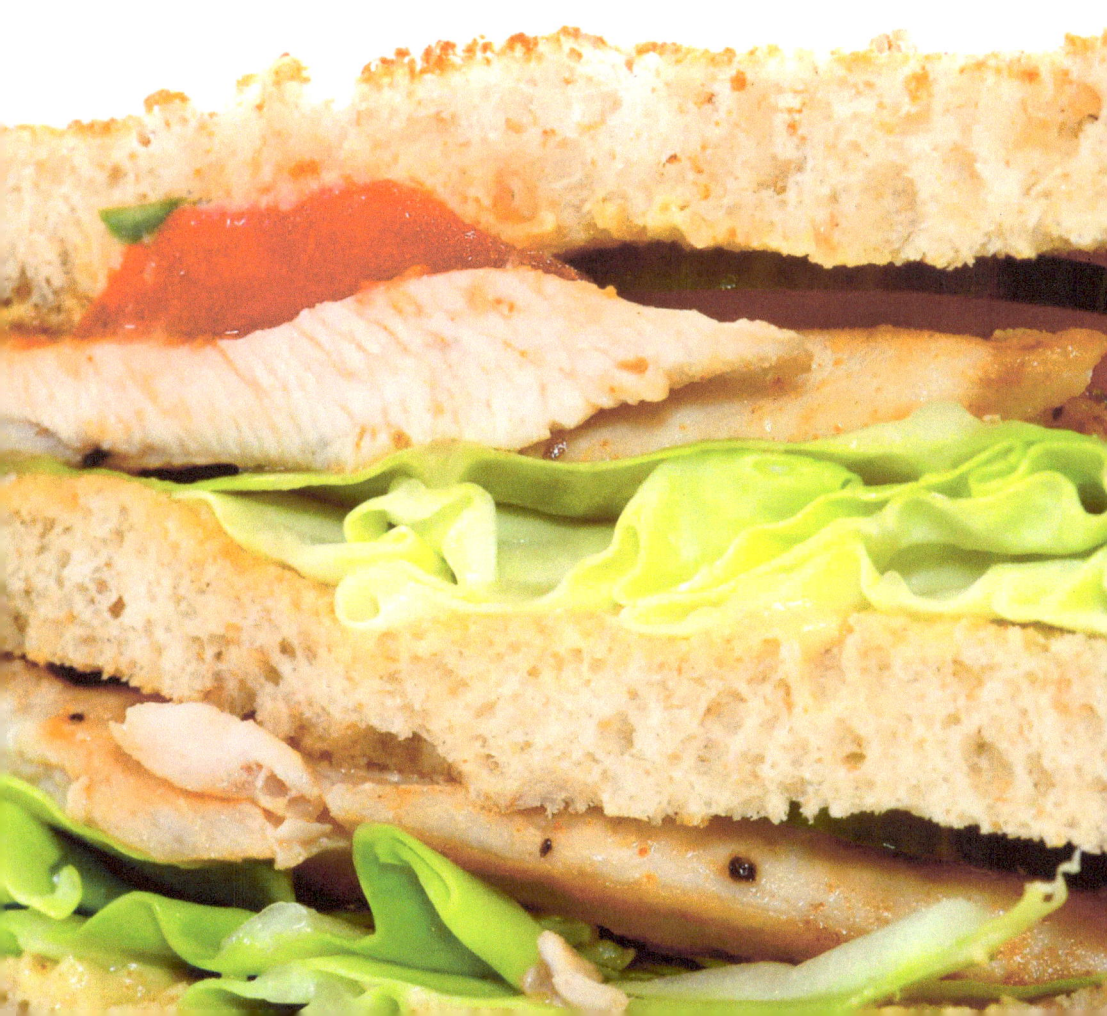

MICRONUTRIENTS

MINERALS

Minerals help our body to function properly because they carry nerve signals, build our bones and clot our blood. They regulate the body's processes and make up body tissues. They keep cells working properly, and can contribute to weight loss. Most of us don't need to supplement with minerals, however a large number of women suffer from iron deficiency. To cope with that lack of iron, it is recommended to take iron supplements. (Consult a specialist to learn more about your optimum mineral supply.)

VITAMINS

Vitamins play a role in our biochemical levels. Their function covers the regulation of the body's biochemical reactions, assist in digestion and use nutrients from various sources. They can be found under two categories: Water-Soluble and Fat-soluble. Water-soluble are Vitamins A, D, E and K. The body natural flushes them out if they are consumed in excessive quantity. (It is visible in the urine color variation.)

On the other hand, your body can build up a large quantity of Fat-Soluble vitamins. Be aware of this information. Don't be tricked by the Bro-scientist spreading wrong or inaccurate DIY multivitamin recipes because Fat-Soluble vitamins can build up and can become harmful at certain levels. To avoid a fat-soluble build up, consult a pharmacist able to recommend a decent multivitamin pill to supplement your food intake.

MICRONUTRIENTS

WATER

Water it is the prime ingredient to any healthy lifestyle. It's divine and the source of life. Water has a pertinent role to play in our lives, fitness level and vitality. It helps in maintaining the body's temperature. It transports nutrients and flushes toxins out from our body. It is absolutely vital to remain and stay hydrated during physical activity. Most importantly, you need to stay hydrated even during inactivity.

It's common knowledge that water is the most abundant liquid present within our bodies. Water contributes up to 70% of our total mass, so remember that you must keep a good water replacement cycle while you release a part of it through the perspiration process. Drink plenty of water to avoid dehydration, keep a sufficient level of water to help your body maintain a fat-burning cycle and a steady nutrient transport in your digestive system.

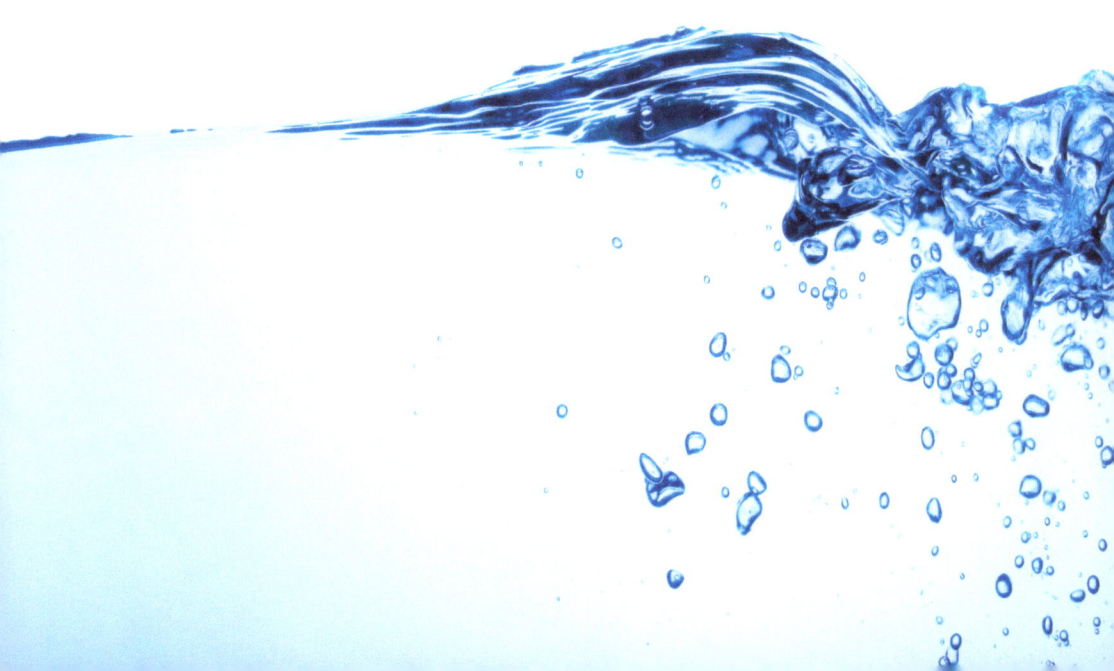

NUTRITION TIPS

A FEW THINGS TO REMEMBER

If sufficient fuel is not added prior to the fat-burning phase, it's better not to skip a meal. The Cardio training will only burn lean muscle tissue to convert it in fat, and destroy some body cells. It's very dangerous to attend a workout with an empty stomach or with a low amount of energy provided by your food intake. Avoid fast and processed foods at all times.

Now with all this knowledge — should you use supplements? Nowadays it's harder to get all our nutrition even with a balanced meal plan. They do strengthen and help to recuperate your body's energy faster. However, I do recommend consulting your physician prior to any supplementation. Medication can conflict with the expected results or completely annihilate the beneficial effects produced by the proper amount of food intake. The most important part in your fitness nutrition plan is the ability to eat in regards of long-term goals. If your goal is to become bigger, you should definitely consider increasing your calorie intake. On the other hand, weight loss requires you to lower a part of your intake to stimulate a fat burning action.

If you want to achieve your best physique and effectively balance your nutritional plan, supplements are recommended — but not mandatory at all. For all of us that need a little boost however, I have included them in this guide. Nowadays, the calorie intake based on the food we eat is not as rich in nutrients as what our grandparents used to eat. We have to admit the fact that most of our food will partially lose a part of the benefits due in part to how we cook it and also the way we prepare it. Supplying your body with the right amount of macronutrients and micronutrients is sometimes a real hassle because we do not have time to select exactly what our metabolism needs according to a specific target weight.

NUTRITION TIPS

Whether your goal is to gain lean mass, lose fat or maintain your current weight, the following supplements come highly recommended:

DIGESTIVE ENZYMES

The digestive enzymes are recommended to help your digestive system break down foods. The enzymes will stimulate and ease the digestion of the proteins, carbohydrates, fats, sugars and dairy. Their function is to provide fast relief from heartburn, gas and bloating, indigestion and more.

FISH OIL

Fish oil will enhance your overall health, skin, brain and joints. It's a real booster that helps to maintain healthy cholesterol and blood pressure, with the ability to reduce the risk of coronary heart disease and support the body's natural anti-inflammatory response.

WHEY PROTEIN

Whey protein is a great source of protein and is quickly digestible making it the perfect choice for a post workout meal. It's also very convenient and extremely flexible in terms of cooking and even baking with protein powders. Whey protein will increase the activation of muscle cells and results in the hypertrophy of the muscles fibers and produces new muscle cells.

NUTRITION TIPS

SHOPPING STRATEGY

Grocery shopping is better with a stomach full of goodness. This is an especially useful tactic to employ that will keep you from feeling that overwhelming hunger as your next grocery store or farmer's market visit. My advice is to re-schedule and avoid temptation. If you have a mean sugar tooth like I do, you'll quickly see the benefit of this practice. Try this trick and feel relief — it's a 100% win.

HEALTHY SHOPPING LIST

CARBOHYDRATES | Oatmeal, Whole Grain Bread, Pitas, Rice (Brown), Pasta, Yams, Apples, Grapefruit, Grapes, Cantaloupe, Strawberries, Plums, Mushrooms, Green Peppers, Broccoli, Tomatoes, Asparagus

PROTEIN | Eggs, Cheese, Ground Beef (10% or less fat), Nonfat Milk, Fresh Turkey, Tuna, Chicken Breast, Sirloin Steak, Low Fat Cottage Cheese

FAT | Eggs, Cheese, Ground Beef (10% or less fat), Nonfat Milk, Raw Nuts, Vegetable Oil, Natural Peanut Butter, Avocado, Olive Oil, Guacamole, Fish Fat, Flax Seed Oil

NUTRITION TIPS

MEAL PLANNING STRATEGY

Plan your meals ahead of time as it will allow you to maximize your food intake. The more muscle you have, the more calories you burn. In order to burn fat, it's required to feed those muscles to burn the excess fat. Building a firm body with toned muscles means that the fat will be used as an energy supply and not be stocked. High metabolism results in "Fat Burning Machine" biomechanics.

ACTIVITY LEVEL

Cardiovascular activity — widely known as aerobic exercise — describes any workout that increases your heart rate, boosts the flow of blood through your body and speeds up your breathing. Biking, walking, jogging, using an elliptical machine, rowing and aerobics are all types of Cardio exercise. Cardio exercises benefit your overall health in many ways.

In addition to reinforcing your cardiovascular system, improving your cardiac strength and keeping your arteries clear, cardio exercise can reduce the risk of serious health problems such as, obesity, heart disease, diabetes, high blood pressure and certain types of cancer. It can also lower the risk of viral illnesses, boost your mood and may even help you live longer and feel better.

Your muscles need energy to work, so the more muscle mass you have, the more calories you burn over the course of the day. It works like this: for every pound of muscle you gain, you will burn 35-50 more calories per day. That doesn't sound like a massive difference, but 15 pounds of muscle instead of fat = 750 calories a day of additional calories burned without even counting your exercise routine. If that isn't a powerful enough reason to start or add a strength-training exercise to your routine, I don't know what is!

NUTRITION TIPS

PORTION SIZING STRATEGY

A quick tip to recreate a balanced meal on the go (if you can't evaluate the amount of food) is to know how to simulate a portion size that complements your macronutrient needs without the chore of weighing food.

PORTION SIZE			
FOOD TYPE	PORTION SIZE	WOMEN	MEN
PROTEIN	Palm of a Hand	1	2
CARBS	Cup of a hand	1	2
FATS / OILS	A thumb	1	2
VEGGIES	A fist	1	2

This practice will provide you with a good reproduction of the food amount to eat without excess. The thickness and density of your meal is not as tricky as you may think. In fact, is almost the same as your hands.

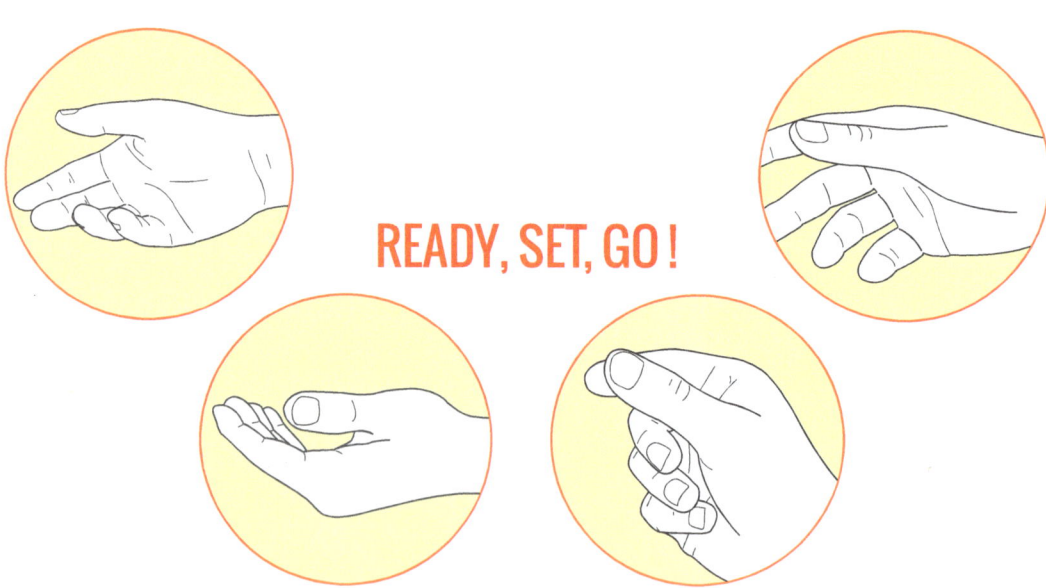

READY, SET, GO !

WHAT IS YOUR BODY TYPE?

There are three general body types — though people tend to share traits and attributes that would land them between the three. A good example would be the Muffin Top, or Flamingo body type. I'm not kidding — they do share traits. Let's see why it's possible and learn a little bit more about the category we fall into. While the ectomorph would be the skinniest frame and also the one with the most contrast, this is something we can also compare to the opposite with a chubby structure, the endomorph. As said previously, many people are a combination of two body types, "Ectomorph / Mesomorph" or "Mesomorph / Endomorph." Be aware of your body's natural response and how your nutrition vibes within you at a physiological level. Start by recognizing which body type is yours. The one that you share the most similarities with, is the body type that you will adjust your meal plan accordingly.

ECTOMORPH

An ectomorph is best described as slender, thin, and skinny. Characteristically, they have delicate bone structure, small shoulders and chest, and a fast metabolism. Ectomorphs are the classic "Hard Gainers." It's very difficult for them to gain weight, as well as put on mass. On the plus side, it's easy for them to get lean. They tend to require a greater percentage of carbohydrates to prevent muscle catabolism, as well as a higher calorie intake overall. Diet Recommendations: Ectomorphs should stick to the high-end range of carbohydrates, (between 30-60 percent of total calories) depending on whether the goal is mass gain, maintenance, or fat loss. Higher carbohydrate ratios increase lean mass gains, while lower carbohydrate ratios tend to accelerate fat loss. It's recommended to stimulate a high-end mass gain to use the mid-upper end for maintenance (45-55 percent), and the low-end for fat loss. At least 25 percent of total calories should come from protein, with the remainder from fat..

MESOMORPH

A mesomorph is someone who trends toward being muscular. They're often strong, athletic hard-body types with well-defined muscles, broad shoulders, and dense bone structure. Mesomorphs generally have little trouble gaining muscle or losing fat, though they will put on fat more readily than ectomorphs. They can handle a moderate level of carbs due to their ample capacity to store muscle glycogen. Weight gain will happen, however, if carbs and calories are exceedingly high. Don't be fooled though — no body type is immune to a bad diet! Diet is the recommendation for Mesomorphs. They do well in the middle range for carbohydrates, between 20-50 percent of total calories. Again, the high-end for mass gains (40-50 percent), the middle for maintenance (30-40), and low-end for fat loss (20-30). To prioritize fat loss, increase both protein and fat while lowering carbohydrate intakes, with no more than 40 percent of calories coming from fat.

ENDOMORPH

The endomorph is best described as soft. They typically have a round or pear-shaped body, shorter limbs, a stocky build, and a slower metabolism. Endomorphs can put on a lot of muscle, but they also tend to carry more adipose tissue and thus have a greater propensity to store fat. Because excess carbohydrates in the endomorph's diet end up as fat, a high carbohydrate intake will make it difficult for them to get lean or lose weight. Their diet recommendations would be to stick to the low end of the carbohydrate range, between 10-40 percent of total calories, depending on their goals. Here, I recommend no more than 30-40 percent carbohydrates for mass gains, the middle range for maintenance (20-30), and low-end for fat loss (10-20). As with the other body types, protein and fat provide the remainder of your calories, with 25-50 percent of total calories from protein and 15-40 percent from fat.

WHAT IS YOUR BODY TYPE?

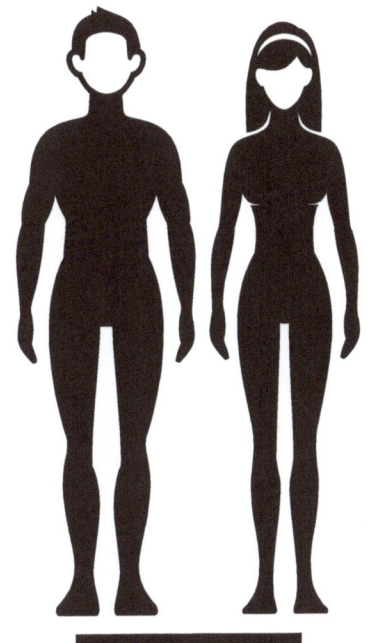

UNDERWEIGHT

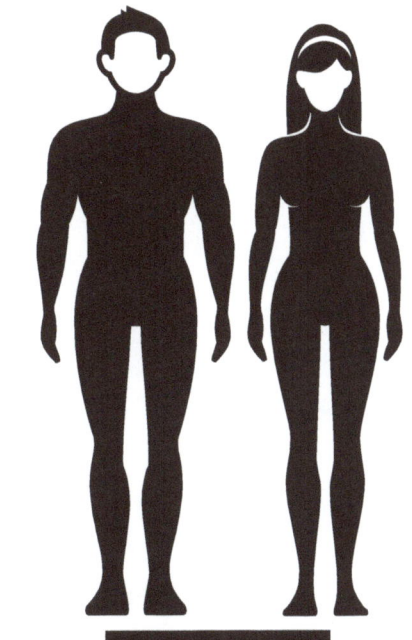

HEALTHY

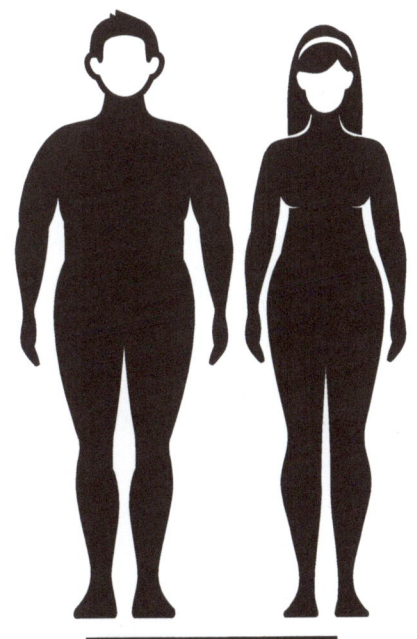

OVERWEIGHT

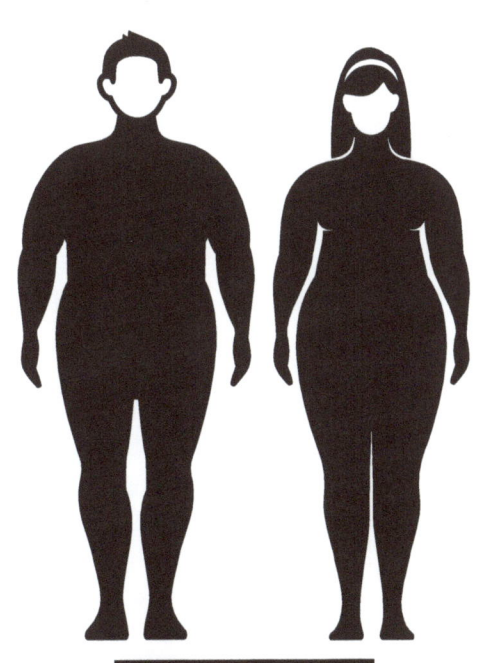

OBESE

Who will have all men to be saved, and to come unto the knowledge of the truth.

- Timothy 2:4

CASE STUDY

I would like to share with you the story of one of my clients. The challenge was to create a concurrent and comprehensive weight loss plan to remotely train her. I was determined to build an effective and powerful outline in order to help my client reach her personal fitness goal. I then found myself reflecting on the following equation while strategizing a plan that directly reflected her body and her fitness goal:

Body composition: 87.7 kg / 193 lbs. (27 year old - female)
Target Weight: 75kg / 165 lbs.
Deadline: 3 Months

THE FOLLOWING IS HER MID-PROGRAM TESTIMONIAL:

"Hello, my name is Bérénice R., and I'm 27 years old. I'm French and currently live in Fairfax. I've known Sébastien for 4 years and this is the first time I'll be working closely with him. My target is to lose 35lbs, have a better body and feel good in my own skin. I remotely follow Sébastien's instruction online. He specifically made a nutrition plan for me and designed a training routine to pair with. It's a pleasure to work with him because he listens to what my problems were in the beginning, I was not able to bend my knees due to past injuries. I have a medical history and it's a chronic condition. As of right now, I can sincerely declare, I feel a true difference. He adapted a training routine for my level and provided a personalized nutrition plan. I truly appreciate his assistance as it not only motivates me, but provides me with an overwhelming source of encouragement. I try to avoid my cravings, but sometimes I did succumb and fell off the program —I like bakery and it's my biggest weakness..."

I want to pinpoint some crucial parts of this testimonial. First, as a team, Bérénice and I went from 87.7kg to 81kg in a month and a half. She was working out at a moderate intensity level for a minimum of 3x/per week. In order to supply her energy level and make sure that her metabolic response would be adequate,

CASE STUDY

I consistently monitored her calorie intake. I have gone to the extent of having her report to me her daily eating habits for our weekly check-in. The process of monitoring food was not easy at first, because she spent most of her life eating according to her appetite rather than her real body needs.

The biggest challenge was to convert those cravings into a healthy eating motion.

There are no magic pills for it; only a realistic method that I am very happy to share with you in my next few sentences. Before we get there, I feel the need to return to the basics of nutrition. I want to make sure that we are on the same page and are fully capable of accurately perceiving our food.

This is why calorie restricted diets are not often sustainable; you are losing lean muscle instead of fat and when you stop the „diet" and gain the weight back, it's not lean muscle.

HOW CAN WE UNDERSTAND CALORIE INTAKE AND NUTRITIONAL FITNESS?

WHAT IS A CALORIE?

First of all, calories are not your enemy or something harmful to you. In fact, calories are necessary to achieve any fitness goal. Whether it's weight loss or to gain lean mass, you need calories! A calorie is a unit of energy. It's the unit we use in nutrition to determine the quality of the food we eat. To elevate the body temperature, the average energy needed to increase the temperature of 1 kilogram of water by 1 °Celsius is 1,000 small calories or approximately 4.2 Kilojoules.

WHY AM I TALKING ABOUT CELSIUS AND KILOJOULES?

It's really simple and has to do with BMR, body heat, the metabolic process and energy production.

IF YOU'RE READY TO HAVE YOUR MIND BLOWN, KEEP READING.

The BMR is also known as the BASAL METABOLIC RATE, and is the number of calories your body needs daily to sustain life. Height, weight, age and gender are used to calculate an individual's BMR.Every time you move or activate your muscles, you burn calories. Yes, I said "burn" — you read correctly.

In order to elevate your body heat and generate energy, your body becomes warm and metabolizes those calories. There are no good or bad calories. They are all converted during special energy production through Metabolic pathways. There are different types of metabolic pathways to convert your calorie intake. However, their main function is to produce the energy needed to create motion.

HOW CAN WE UNDERSTAND CALORIE INTAKE AND NUTRITIONAL FITNESS?

DO YOU GET MY POINT NOW?

NO CALORIES = NO ENERGY

MIND BLOWING, ISN'T IT?

Now is the time to keep up that excellent focus! Let's get more specific with an example: I am on a diet and my goal is to lose fat.

WHICH OF THE FOLLOWING WILL HELP ME REACH MY GOAL?

1. Try a low-carb diet

2. Stop and avoid eating fat at all costs

3. Ask my mom to stop cooking at home (Sorry Mom)

4. Run on an empty stomach 3x/week

5. Only eat protein

6. Eat more.

YES, I KNOW YOU THINK I'M CRAZY...

How is it possible to lose weight by eating more? It's simple: remember the BMR calculation. Imagine that I need 2000 calories a day to be healthy. If I don't work out and only eat a small portion of food with reduced fat throughout the day, by the time I go to sleep my calorie intake has reached 1870 calories

HOW CAN WE UNDERSTAND CALORIE INTAKE AND NUTRITIONAL FITNESS?

WILL I LOSE WEIGHT?

Well, hmm... yes, but at what cost? I just dropped some weight unexpectedly. I don't understand what happened. I should be happy, but I'm beginning to feel weak, dizzy and tired.

Oh, no! I lost lean body mass!!!

ARE CALORIES MONSTERS?

Number 2, 3... Nope, you are close. It's Number 6.

The right answer is 6.

Yep, that's the tricky part. If you don't help your body to burn fat, it will automatically select an easier portion of your body to breakdown in order to produce energy. The lean body mass (aka, those muscles that I hardly build at the gym) are in a critical process called the catabolic phase. Since I did not provide a sufficient amount of calories to protect them, the natural body reaction is to burn muscle instead of fat. Now you know that reducing my calorie intake below 2000 was a huge mistake.

Most importantly, I was not even working out. I virtually starved my body of a vital component and let my body take drastic measures to allow me to recover. If I did workout, I could have been in an even more dangerous situation.

If I really want to lose that unwanted fat, I NEED TO EAT MORE FOOD!

HOW CAN WE UNDERSTAND CALORIE INTAKE AND NUTRITIONAL FITNESS?

WHY?

That's easy.

THE BODY NEEDS A SUPERIOR AMOUNT OF CALORIES TO CREATE ENERGY AND BURN FAT INSTEAD OF MY DEAR, LEAN MUSCLE-MASS.

How could we run, lift, or jump without energy provided by that lovely food? The body burns calories during your sleep too... That's why you are starving before your breakfast. Yes, my friend, you were fasting all night long! Go get yourself some food and start the day with a belly full of nutrients. Help yourself by giving it the fuel to metabolize and break down fat.

Eat enough in order to be on the positive side of the scale! You will maintain lean mass, drop that fat and become toned, energetic and most importantly, feel sexier and more attractive than ever!

Stop being afraid of the Calorie Monster and kick it in the butt. You are in control. Nothing can get in your way when you're on the amazing and rewarding journey to positive fitness and health.

RECOMMENDED FOOD LIST

Bananas

Contain 23 grams of carbohydrates per 3 ½ ounces, a low amount of protein, and less than 1 gram of fat. It's a good source of potassium, vitamin B6, vitamin C and magnesium

Beans

Contain nearly no fat and are a rich source of vitamin B6 and B12. Potassium, zinc, calcium, iron and magnesium are also benefits provided by beans. They are made of about 25% of protein and a good supply of carbohydrates. Their digestion is slow which provides a steady energy release.

Beans

Contain nearly no fat and are a rich source of vitamin B6 and B12. Potassium, zinc, calcium, iron and magnesium are also benefits provided by beans. They are made of about 25% of protein and a good supply of carbohydrates. Their digestion is slow which provides a steady energy release.

Broccoli

Broccoli contains about 30 calories, 1 gram of fat, 5 grams of carbohydrates and 3 grams of protein per 3 ½ ounces serving. It also contains vitamin C, calcium folate, vitamin B6, manganese, potassium and beta-carotene.

Carrots

We all know carrots are good for our eyesight – but why? Carrots are very high in vitamin A, which is responsible for proper functioning of the retina. They contain very little fat and a modest amount of protein, while also very rich in carbohydrates, vitamin C and potassium. If you enjoy eating them raw, remember to always clean your carrots thoroughly with a vegetable brush to avoid consuming bacteria that may have built up.

Egg whites

Egg whites are packed with pure protein. They're considered nearly perfect because of their sublime blend of amino acids. The white of one egg contains four grams of pure protein. This is the cheapest and best protein you could ever consume.

RECOMMENDED FOOD LIST

Oatmeal

Oatmeal is a tremendous source of high quality carbohydrates. It has more protein than wheat, twice as much as brown rice, and is very low in fat. The total amount of fat is less than 2 grams per serving, which is hardly enough fat intake to worry about. Oatmeal is a good source of iron and manganese, and has high amounts of vitamin E, copper, folate and zinc. It's a great source of dietary fiber and it helps lower cholesterol. As an inexpensive pre-workout meal ingested one hour before training, oatmeal also makes a superior energy source for a tough workout.

Pasta

Pasta is virtually fat free if eaten by itself, so forget about the fat-filled sauces, sausages and meatballs. Use vegetable-rich tomato-based sauces instead. Pasta contains less than 1 gram of fat and about 2 grams of protein for every 3 ½ ounces. It's rich in vitamin B6, magnesium and copper. Go for a whole-grain variety.

Sweet Potatoes

Most people assume that because of their sweet taste, sweet potatoes are higher in calories than regular potatoes. This isn't true. An enzyme in sweet potatoes converts starches into sugars and this adds to the deliciously sweet taste. Every 3 ½ ounces contains 2 grams of protein, 24 grams of carbohydrates, and an adequate amount of dietary fiber and less than 1 gram of fat. They're also rich in vitamin A, vitamin C and vitamin B6 along with traces of copper and magnesium.

Tuna

Tuna is particularly convenient and very high in protein with 30 grams of protein per 3 ½ ounce servings and less than 1 gram of fat. Tuna also contains 100 percent of the RDA for B12, and is a rich source of niacin, phosphorus, vitamin B6, magnesium and potassium. Albacore, bluefin and yellowfin are the three types of tuna most commonly found fresh or canned.

Turkey

Turkey breast is the leanest of any meat (without the skin of course). A 3 ½ ounce serving contains 1 gram of fat and 30 grams of protein. It contains high amounts of vitamin B12 and B6, copper, iron, niacin, phosphorus, riboflavin and zinc.

FRUITS AND VEGGIES

FRUIT/VEGGIES	BENEFITS
APPLES	Protects your heart, Prevents constipation, Blocks diarrhea, Improves lung capacity, Cushions joints
APRICOTS	Combats cancer, Controls blood pressure, Saves your eyesight, Shields against Alzheimer's, Slows aging process
ARTICHOKES	Aids digestion, Lowers cholesterol, Protects your heart, Stabilizes blood sugar, Guards against liver disease
AVOCADOS	Battles diabetes, Lowers cholesterol, Helps stops strokes, Controls blood pressure, Smoothes skin
BANANAS	Protects your heart, Quiets a cough, Strengthens bones, Controls blood pressure, Blocks diarrhea
BEANS	Prevents constipation, Helps hemorrhoids, Lowers cholesterol, Combats cancer, Stabilizes blood sugar
BEETS	Controls blood pressure, Combats cancer, Strengthens bones, Protects your heart, Aids weight loss
BLUEBERRIES	Combats cancer, Protects your heart, Stabilizes blood sugar, Boosts memory, Prevents constipation
BROCCOLI	Strengthens bones, Saves eyesight, Combats cancer, Protects your heart, Controls blood pressure
CABBAGE	Combats cancer, Prevents constipation, Promotes weight loss, Protects your heart, Helps hemorrhoids
CANTALOUPE	Saves eyesight, Controls blood pressure, Lowers cholesterol, Combats cancer, Supports immune system
CARROTS	Saves eyesight, Protects your heart, Prevents constipation, Combats cancer, Promotes weight loss
CAULIFLOWER	Protects against Prostate Cancer, Combats Breast Cancer, Strengthens bones, Banishes bruises, Guards against heart
CHERRIES	Protects your heart, Combats Cancer, Ends insomnia, Slows aging process, Shields against
CHESTNUTS	Promotes weight loss, Protects your heart, Lowers cholesterol, Combats Cancer, Controls blood pressure
CHILI PEPPERS	Aids digestion, Soothes sore throat, Clears sinuses, Combats Cancer, Boosts immune system
FIGS	Promotes weight loss, Helps stops strokes, Lowers cholesterol, Combats Cancer, Controls blood pressure
FLAX SEEDS	Aids digestion, Battles diabetes, Protects your heart, Improves mental health, Boosts immune system
GARLIC	Lowers cholesterol, Controls blood pressure, Combats cancer, Kills bacteria, Fights fungus
GRAPEFRUIT	Protects against heart attacks, Promotes Weight loss, Helps stops strokes, Combats Prostate Cancer, Lowers cholesterol
GRAPES	Saves eyesight, Conquers kidney stones, Combats cancer, Enhances blood flow, Protects your heart
GREEN TEA	Combats cancer, Protects your heart, Helps stops strokes, Promotes Weight loss, Kills bacteria
HONEY	Heals wounds, Aids digestion, Guards against ulcers, Increases energy, Fights allergies
LEMONS	Combats cancer, Protects your heart, Controls blood pressure, Smoothes skin, Stops scurvy
LIMES	Combats cancer, Protects your heart, Controls blood pressure, Smoothes skin, Stops scurvy
MANGOES	Combats cancer, Boosts memory, Regulates thyroid, Aids digestion, Shields against Alzheimer's

FRUITS AND VEGGIES

FRUIT/VEGGIES	BENEFITS
MUSHROOMS	Controls blood pressure, Lowers cholesterol, Kills bacteria, Combats cancer, Strengthens bones
OATS	Lowers cholesterol, Combats cancer, Battles diabetes, Prevents constipation, Smoothes skin
OLIVE OIL	Protects your heart, Promotes Weight loss, Combats cancer, Battles diabetes, Smoothes skin
ONIONS	Reduce risk of heart attack, Combats cancer, Kills bacteria, Lowers cholesterol, Fights fungus
ORANGES	Supports immune systems, Combats cancer, Protects your heart, Straightens respiration
PEACHES	Prevents constipation, Combats cancer, Helps stops strokes, Aids digestion, Helps hemorrhoids
PINEAPPLE	Strengthens bones, Relieves colds, Aids digestion, Dissolves warts, Blocks diarrhea
PRUNES	Slows aging process, Prevents constipation, Boosts memory, Lowers cholesterol, Protects against heart disease
STRAWBERRIES	Combats cancer, Protects your heart, Boosts memory, Calms stress
SWEET POTATO-ES	Saves your eyesight, Lifts mood, Combats cancer, Strengthens bones
TOMATOES	Protects prostate, Combats cancer, Lowers cholesterol, Protects your heart
WALNUTS	Lowers cholesterol, Combats cancer, Boosts memory, Lifts mood, Protects against heart disease
WATERMELON	Protects prostate, Promotes Weight loss, Lowers cholesterol, Helps stops strokes, Controls blood pressure
WHEAT GERM	Combats Colon Cancer, Prevents constipation, Lowers cholesterol, Helps stops strokes, improves digestion
WHEAT BRAN	Combats Colon Cancer, Prevents constipation, Lowers cholesterol, Helps stops strokes, improves digestion

HOW DO WE AVOID CRAVINGS?

A FEW THINGS TO REMEMBER

If you experience the need to eat a specific type of food, it means that you are missing an essential element in your nutritional plan. The best manner to counter that craving is to determine what you are missing. Once you know what you need, it will be easier to react with a healthy response and the proper behavior. Breaking through bad eating habits is not something to take lightly. This is why I want to give you an example and explain what you can do to avoid going back and forth to the fridge and eating with guilt. The chart below will help you to pinpoint what is preventing you from satisfying your appetite. Try to remember that it's always better to ingest the nutrient based on real food first. If for any reasons there is a need to supplement in another manner, be sure to prioritize solid food, liquid, then supplement. Do not cut or eliminate anything your body naturally makes to digest. What you need is to supply your body with energy with your daily calorie intake. You don't want to put your body in a potentially negative state and mess up your organs.

I'm craving...	I truly Need	What are my food Alternatives?
Chocolate	Magnesium	Nuts, Seeds, Legumes, Fruit
Sugary Food, Sweets	Chromium	Broccoli, Grapes, Cheese, Chicken
	Carbon	Fresh Fruit
	Phosphorus	Chicken, Beef, Fish, Eggs, Dairy, Nuts, Legumes, Grains
	Sulfur	Cranberries, Horseradish, Cauliflower, Broccoli, Cabbage
	Tryptophan	Cheese, Lamb, Liver, Raisins, Sweet Potato, Spinach
Bread, Toast, Pasta, Carbs	Nitrogen	High Protein Foods: Meat, Fish, Nuts, Beans
Oily/Fatty Foods	Calcium	Milk, Cheese, Yoghurt, Legumes, Broccoli, Green Leafy Vegetables
Salty Foods	Chloride	Fish, Goat's Milk
	Silicon	Nuts, Seeds; (except unrefined starches)

GLUTEN FREE, FAT FREE, LIGHT, 0%

You're probably wondering what all those words and labels are about. Well you're in luck — this chart will help you in your food selection process while doing your groceries. Most of us just follow the big trends and buy food based solely on the idea that it's good according to the quality/taste value. Many go as far as ignoring carcinogenic (cancer causing) ingredients such as BHA and some artificial food coloring, all for the sake of momentary pleasure when eating. In a weight loss nutrition plan made without enough knowledge, its way too easy to give in on our grocery trip. Light soda, 0% yogurt, low fat this, fat free that. I want to stop you right there. Don't get fooled again. You want to ensure that you're creating a pleasant tasting experience and something as close to normal, healthy eating as possible. The unfortunate truth is the food you eat is worked, or modified to reproduce a similar flavor. How many labels managed to ensnare you with their empty promises of, „No sugar added, sugar free, low blah blah..."

Did you ever realize all the things needed to make something tasty sits right at the pinnacle of natural, organic food components? What happens when you remove every last bit of natural semblance in your meal? It becomes a time-bomb in your body. Yes, it's that bad. Wait, that's not the worst part. Think of your protein intake. When you get your protein from animal protein previously jacked up for mass production, does your body, or more specifically, your digestive system get affected by it? Yes, because the antibiotic and/or chemicals being eaten from your food are playing a very big role in transforming your body into something it's not. After all, your body can hardly recognize the junk you put in your mouth as "food", so it doesn't understand what to do with it and that can cause serious problems in and of itself.

Think of that before buying food next time. Carefully examine what you will be consuming before you purchase. I know that organic foods are a little more pricey compared to the food we first see on display, but it is worth the price. You are extending your lifespan. All of this has been to remind you of one thing. You and I are what we eat. Yes, my friends. We are reaching a time period that will be decisive for our future as human beings. Some will become weaker because the foods they have eaten have made them prone to illness, coupled with poor lifestyle choices. Others will become stronger with an increase in their

GLUTEN FREE, FAT FREE, LIGHT, 0%

metabolism response resulting in an appropriate calorie intake. Quality prevails over quantity and the choices you made in your past might become a blueprint of what your overall health will display for your future. Let's try to be righteous from the start.

I want to address one thing that stands out to me regarding the Gluten Freak. I am still able to eat food that contains gluten. I was originally against the gluten free movement at first because I have a general resistance to things that are not mastered. Unless people tell me the truth behind it, I will strongly ask and even command a more elaborate answer. I have done my research and put my name on the line.

I can now tell you why I believe in this current movement. As long as it produces positive health with no harmful counterparts, I will continue to be its proponent. Until I see major objections to modify the food selection, it will continue to be a specially crafted, beneficial guide to follow. Since food companies are always trying to take advantage of the dietary trend or health craze, it's important to arm yourself with this knowledge.

Take this opportunity to be in the loop. Break away from being that simple consumer that purchases blindly from major corporations that care more about saving a dollar than how their dangerous ingredients are affecting society's overall health. Update yourself with knowledge on the topic.

GLUTEN FREE, FAT FREE, LIGHT, 0%

Gluten free food can be found in these categories:

- Beans, seeds, nuts in their natural, unprocessed form
- Fresh eggs, Fresh meats, fish and poultry (not breaded, batter-coated or marinated)
- Fruits and vegetables and also most dairy products

Most people with Gluten intolerance will notice right away if they are having trouble digesting foods which contain gluten, so eating Gluten-Free food can help them avoid potential digestive suffering and complications, and maintain a healthy lifestyle.

Again, this is my take and you are free to agree with me or not. Still, I want you to be aware that there are a lot of processed Gluten-Free products that are on the market, which still contain high dosages of other ingredients, like sugar, high fructose corn syrup, caramel coloring, and other depleting ingredients. So, again, just as I mentioned with the „diet" and „low fat" labels, just because it says „Gluten-Free" doesn't mean it's the best and healthiest option for your optimum vitality.

Go, eat your food with gladness, and drink your wine with a joyful heart, for it is now that God favors what you do.

- Ecclesiastes 9:7

MEALS & SMOOTHIES

CLEAN AND LEAN

If your goal is to remain in the best shape, a balanced meal is what you need. Don't miss this opportunity to enjoy yourself while trying these healthy, filling, and clean recipes full of the best nutrients for your body.

POP'S WAFFLE

Ingredients:

1/3 cups of flour

4 teaspoons of baking powder

½ teaspoon of salt

2 teaspoons of sugar

2 eggs separated

½ cup of clarified butter (melted)

¾ cup of milk

Directions:

In a large mixing bowl, whisk together all dry ingredients. Separate the eggs, adding the yolk to the dry ingredient mixture and placing the whites in a small mixing bowl. Beat whites until moderately stiff then set aside. Add milk and melted butter to dry ingredient mixture and blend. Fold stiff egg whites into mixture. Pour mixture into hot waffle iron and bake.

MEALS & SMOOTHIES

WHITE OMELETTE

Ingredients:

4 organic egg whites

2 tablespoons water

1 tablespoon clarified butter or cooking spray.

1 clove of garlic

1 pinch of sea salt

1 Provence herbs or Persil (for hint)

Shredded cheese (optional)

Directions:

Crack 4 eggs and separate the yolk. Beat the whites with a fork, then add a teaspoon of oil. While beating the ingredients together add 1 pinch of sea salt. The next step is to prepare the seasoning. Pour the water in a small cup, and chop the garlic clove into thin pieces and add to the cup with the Persil. Mix it gently and whisk all ingredients together. Cook the mixture and keep the stove on low. When the omelette starts to have bubbles on the top, it is almost ready to be folded or flipped. If you prefer to add cheese, feel free to evenly distribute some shredded cheese to the top or inside your folded omelette.

MEALS & SMOOTHIES

TURKEY BALLS

Ingredients:

1 lb. of ground turkey breast
½ cup of ground flax seeds
¼ cup of wheat bran cereal
½ small onion chopped
2 beaten egg whites
salt & pepper

Directions:

Mix all the ingredients together in a large bowl, then separate into 2 inch meatballs and place on a cookie sheet coated with olive oil or cooking spray. Bake at 375 degrees Fahrenheit for about 30 minutes. Meatballs are ready to eat when an inserted fork comes out clean.

PASTA AND GREENS

Ingredients:

125g of pasta
1 organic beaten egg
20g of butter
½ cup of cream
½ cup of grated Parmesan
1 bunch asparagus trimmed, halved and blanched
Snipped chives and salad to serve

Directions:

Cook the 125g of pasta in a large saucepan of boiling and salted water. After the pasta is cooked, drain the pasta and return to pan. Add 1 beaten egg, 20g of butter, ½ cup of cream and grated Parmesan to the pasta. Toss it quickly over a low heat. Add 1 bunch trimmed, halved and blanched asparagus. Serve the plate topped with snipped chives and accompany with salad.

MEALS & SMOOTHIES

TRI-CHOCO TASTY BAR

Ingredients:

4-6 scoops of whey protein (vanilla flavor)
¼ cup of chocolate chips (Milk chocolate/White chocolate/Dark chocolate)
½ cup of rice crispy cereal
1 tablespoon of vanilla extract
½ tablespoon of salted butter
½ cup of water
½ cup of sugar powder

Directions:

In a large bowl combine the whey, chocolate chips, and salted butter. Mix completely: press into an 8x8 inch baking dish coated with olive oil cooking spray. The dough will be very sticky, so the best method for spreading evenly into the baking dish is to use two large spoons coated with olive oil cooking spray. Push the bottom of the spoons onto the dough and push them in opposite directions, until the dough is spread evenly.

Just before baking, press the puffed rice cereal into the top of the dough. Do not mix Rice Crispy into the dough earlier, or they will become soggy and lose their crisp.

Bake at 350-degrees Fahrenheit for 10 minutes.

MEALS & SMOOTHIES

BUFF AND STUFF

Always wondered how to build a strong frame, rock hard muscles or even just supply the sufficient energy in your body to keep yourself at the top of your fitness level? Here we go! A real meal that will turn you into a hero who is ready to protect and serve follows.

MUM'S CREPES

Ingredients:

1 cup of skim milk

2 ounces of butter

3 organic eggs

4 ounces of flour

1 ounce of sugar

1 pinch of salt

A few drops of vanilla extract, rum, etc. (optional)

Preparation:

About 8 large crepes or 12 small.

Directions:

Start the preparation by melting the butter and mix with the milk. Then take a few minutes to let it cool down. Beat the 3 eggs with a fork. Add the beaten eggs into the bowl of flour then add the sugar and a pinch of salt. Mix these ingredients until smooth. Then, take the milk with the melted butter and pour it slowly into the bowl with the other ingredients while still beating the mixture.

MEALS & SMOOTHIES

If you would like to give a special aroma to the crepes, feel free to incorporate vanilla extract, rum etc. You're your opportunity to be creative and adjust the recipe to your specific preferences!

Your crepe batter is now ready for the stove! Here is my personal trick: If the batter seems to be too thick for your taste, beat it before spreading it onto the pan with a tablespoon of oil. It will make your crepes moist and you'll be a pro at air-flipping them!

MEALS & SMOOTHIES

POWER SMASHED DOUGH

Ingredients:

Crust:

½ cup of whole wheat flour

1 cup of wheat bran cereal

¼ teaspoon of baking powder

¼ teaspoon of salt

½ cup of water

Toppers:

½ lb. of 96% lean ground beef or chicken

1 small onion chopped

2 cloves of garlic

1 cup of chopped mushrooms

1 large tomato diced

1 large green pepper chopped

½ cup of shredded mozzarella

Basil and Oregano to taste

Hot Sauce (optional)

Directions:

Mix the crust ingredients together in a large bowl. Then place into a 9x12-inch pan, spreading the crust 1-inch up the side of the pan. Bake the crust by itself in the oven at 400-degrees Fahrenheit for five minutes.

In a large skillet, stir-fry the ground beef and garlic for 3 minutes until beef or chicken starts to brown. Add the chopped onions, mushrooms, tomatoes, and green peppers to the stir-fry for an additional 3 minutes. Transfer the meat and vegetables to the baking dish/pan, and spread evenly over the crust. Top it with shredded mozzarella, and bake at 400-degrees a Fahrenheit for 12 minutes. Use broil setting for the last 4 minutes.

MEALS & SMOOTHIES

ENTANGLED SALMON

Ingredients:
100g of spaghetti
125g of broccoli
50 tablespoons of Philadelphia light cooking crème
50g of smoked chopped salmon
2 teaspoons of lemon zest, finely grated
2 teaspoons of baby capers and dill

Directions:
Begin to cook the spaghetti in a large pan of boiling salted water. Once the pasta is almost al dente, add broccoli. Cover and return to boil, then uncover and cook until ready. Drain and return to the pan. Add cream, salmon, lemon zest, capers and dill. Toss to combine and heat through. Season to taste and serve immediately.

TASTY PASTA & TUNA

Ingredients:
50g penne pasta
2 peeled, julienned carrots
2 julienned, seeded cucumbers
80g drained and flaked spring-water tuna
2 tablespoons of snipped chives
½ cup light sour cream
½ cup sweet chili sauce
1 tablespoon of olive oil

Directions:
Cook the penne in a pan with salted boiling water. When al dente, drain pasta and allow it to cool. Add carrots, cucumbers, tuna and chives to the penne. Mix the sour cream and chili sauce in a small mixing bowl. Then add to this to the penne mixture and toss to combine.

MEALS & SMOOTHIES

EVERYBODY'S CHICKEN

Ingredients:

2 pieces of chicken breast

25g cubed and steamed pumpkin

25g cubed and steamed carrots

50g fennel, diced and sautéed in olive oil

1 lemon juice

¼ cup of pine nuts

1 tablespoon of fresh chopped sage

1 tablespoon of olive oil

Directions:

Preheat oven to 180 degrees Celsius. Place all of the steamed and chopped ingredients except the chicken, into a bowl and add olive oil to help mix well until you have a pasta consistency. Place the chicken breast on a chopping board and carefully cut a pocket into the breast. Use your hands to push the mixture/stuffing into the pocket that you cut and then bring the flap back over and place the chicken breast face down. Close with a toothpick or skewers if needed. Place on a baking tray in the oven and cook until chicken is cooked through and is golden brown on both sides. Serve with rice and steamed vegetables.

MEALS & SMOOTHIES

FRESH AND GREEN

Do you remember what mom always said? "Sweetie, eat your veggies." To continue making our dear mothers happy, let's try to cook the tastiest homemade salad with ingredients your mom would be proud of! Let's make it sweet, spicy, salty and don't forget yummy!

PATRA'S PRIDE

Ingredients:

1 large chopped cucumber

1 large diced red tomato

1 tablespoon of olive oil

1 freshly diced onion

Dash of salt & pepper

Diced feta cheese (optional)

Directions:

Chop the cucumber and tomato into small cubes, then toss with the olive oil, salt and pepper. Serve chilled.

MEALS & SMOOTHIES

TUNA SANDWICH

Ingredients:

12 ounce chunky tuna

2 white onions (minced)

2 tablespoons of black mustard seeds

2 beaten organic eggs

1 tablespoon of Provence herbs

2 cloves of garlic chopped

2 teaspoons of olive oil

salt & pepper to taste

Directions:

Combine all of the ingredients except olive oil in a large bowl. Form into two large patties. Drizzle the olive oil in a skillet. Then pan fry the tuna blend in the skillet over medium heat for about 6 minutes on each side, until both sides are browned and the patties are cooked through.

MEALS & SMOOTHIES

BARBECUE MINIZZA

Ingredients:

2 x 15cm pizza bases
50g of beef minced
50g of chicken minced
½ cup of barbecue sauce
2 cups of grated mozzarella cheese
1 chopped tomato
1 sliced red onion
parsley for topping
salt & pepper to taste
Chili flakes (optional)

Directions:

Preheat oven to hot, (200°C.) Slightly grease 2 baking trays, line with baker paper. Heat 2 teaspoons olive oil in a small frying pan on high. Brown 50g mince beef and chicken for about 5 minutes. Place the 2 pizza bases on prepared tray, spread1/2 cup barbecues sauce evenly then added 1 slice tomato and onion with the grate mozzarella between them. Bake for 12-15 minutes until cheese melts and is lightly browned. Sprinkle with parsley. (chili flakes). Cut into wedges and serve immediately

MEALS & SMOOTHIES

SPICY CHICKEN & AVOCADO

Ingredients:
3 peeled and chopped red-skinned potatoes
¼ cup of milk (warm)
20g of butter
1 teaspoon of coriander
1 teaspoon of cumin
½ teaspoon of paprika
1 tablespoon of olive oil
2 chicken breast fillets
50g of baby rocket leaves
1 tablespoon of extra virgin olive oil
1 chopped avocado
1 juiced lemon
2 teaspoons of horseradish cream

Directions:
Cook the potatoes in a large pot of boiling salted water for 10-15 minutes until tender. Drain and return to the pot, then mash them well. Add milk and butter and continue to mash until smooth. In a small mixing bowl mix together coriander, cumin, paprika and one teaspoon of olive oil. Then rub seasoning all over the chicken breast. Heat the remaining olive oil in a non-stick frying pan on medium heat. Cook the chicken for 4-5 minutes on each side until cooked through, and let it rest for 5 minutes.

Place avocado, lemon juice and horseradish cream in a blender. Blend until smooth, then transfer to a bowl. Add 1/3 cup of water and stir together to make the avocado dressing.

Slice the chicken into thick strips and lay them over. Then spoon over the avocado dressing and drizzle with extra virgin olive oil. Serve with a side of mashed potatoes on the plate. Enjoy!

MEALS & SMOOTHIES

BEEF WRAPS

Ingredients:

1 diced tomato

½ red onion finely chopped

1 tablespoon of coriander

2 wholegrain wraps (or pita bread)

3 iceberg lettuce leaves (shredded)

3 roast beef slices cut into strips

½ cup grated cheese

Directions:

Combine tomatoes, onions and coriander in a small bowl and season to taste. Lay out the wraps, then top with lettuce and sliced roast beef. Then sprinkle with cheese, and spoon some of the tomato salsa on top. Roll up to enclose.

MEALS & SMOOTHIES

SMOOTHIE AND CREAM

Enjoy these five delightful and delicious shakes and smoothies. They're a wonderful "on-the-go" alternative to keep your body nourished between meals. Each one takes 45 seconds to make and provides you with healthy eating benefits.

ESSENCE OF MELI

Ingredients:

1 cup of low-fat milk

2 scoops of protein powder (or two raw eggs)

1 tablespoon of honey

½ banana

2 scoops of vanilla ice cream

Ice cubes (optional)

Directions:

Use a blender to mix the ingredients and get ready to taste a real power surge. It can be taken as an alternative breakfast or a post-workout shake depending on the protein powder included in the mixture.

MEALS & SMOOTHIES

EVERGREEN HARMONY

Ingredients:

2 cups of purified spring water

1 freshly squeezed lemon

1 freshly squeezed lime

1 kiwi

½ cup of celery

1 pineapple

1 cucumber

1 kale

Ginger (optional pinch of ginger)

Directions:

Combine the above ingredients in a blender to produce an average of 10 ounces per serving.

GOLDEN ORB INFUSION

Ingredients:

2 cups of purified spring water

2 freshly squeezed lemons

1-2 pinches of organic cayenne pepper

1-2 tablespoons of organic maple syrup or raw organic non-pasteurized honey

1 cube of brown sugar

Directions:

Combine the ingredients in a blender to produce an average of 10 ounces drink per serving.

MEALS & SMOOTHIES

VANILLA FROST

Ingredients:

½ banana

2 cups of French vanilla ice cream

1 tablespoon of vanilla extract

1 pinch of cannelle

1 cup of skim milk (or almond milk)

1 scoop of whey-protein

Directions:

Blend and combine everything for about 60 sec in the blender. Consistency and thickness may vary depending on your personal preference and on the amount of milk added to the mix..

SCARLET MIST

Ingredients:

1 banana

1 cup of strawberries

1 cup of raspberry

1 cup of skim milk

1 scoop of whey-protein

1 cup of ice cream (strawberry flavor)

Directions:

Blend and combine everything for about 60 sec in the blender. Consistency and thickness may vary depending on your personal preference and on the amount of milk added to the mix.

CONCLUSION

Thank you for taking this journey with me and giving me the opportunity to teach you more about nutrition. Be proud of yourself! You have taken a large step in the right direction to achieving your fitness goals. To conclude, I would like to leave you with some imperative advice: Always remember that Fitness and Nutrition go hand in hand. The quality of your progress and energy level is directly related to your daily food intake. After each meal, your body experiences an immediate change in metabolism. Prepare your meals in advance and take those little steps today, which will make a huge difference in the long run.

You must eat as much fresh food as possible. Eat 6-8 servings of vegetables per day, try new ways to cook them and never get bored. Enjoy their benefits by including them into your meals. Fruit can be eaten all day long, use them too. They are not harmful to you achieving your goal; in fact it's quite the opposite.

Do not hesitate to write down a list before going grocery shopping in order to keep track of healthy foods to buy and avoid becoming a victim of your cravings.

Do not underestimate the value provided by the different sources of fibers comprised in your diet. Vitamins are good for your body. High quality, low-fat protein such as egg whites, and low-fat or fat-free milks, should be a priority in your protein sources.

Fat is already present is your food — this is the reason why you can allow yourself to focus on the type of carbohydrates and proteins you will eat with ease. Try to Limit or remove the usage of salt during the cooking process. Most of the food we eat is already high in sodium. Avoid sodas and beverages that are very rich in

CONCLUSION

sugar.Read the labels. If the ingredient list is long or you can't pronounce most of the ingredients listed, odds are it may not be as healthy (or close to real food) as the label suggests.

On that note, I invite you to try the recipes I shared with you. Expand your kitchen adventures with your own ingredients and variations. Make it as tasty and close to your personal liking.

This guide is here to help you to look at food as an ally and not something to fear. I truly hope that this book was helpful to you and has made you eager to learn more. It will be a pleasure to provide you with even more knowledge in my next book to come.

Sébastien Leria

HIIT WORKOUT

HERMES' RUN

Pain / Minutes	Speed (Mph)	Mount Olympus Incline (%)
00:00 - 00:01	6	3%
00:01 - 00:02	6	6%
00:02 - 00:03	8	8%
00:03 - 00:04	10	7%
00:04 - 00:05	12	6%
00:05 - 00:06	14	5%
00:06 - 00:07	8	8%
00:07 - 00:08	10	7%
00:08 - 00:09	12	6%
00:09 - 00:10	14	5%
00:10 - 00:11	8	8%
00:11 - 00:12	10	7%
00:12 - 00:13	12	6%
00:13 - 00:14	14	5
00:14 - 00:15	8	8%
00:15 - 00:16	10	7%
00:16 - 00:17	12	6%
00:17 - 00:18	14	5%
00:18 - 00:19	6	3%
00:19 - 00:20	2	1%

20 MINUTES OF CARDIO-TORMENT

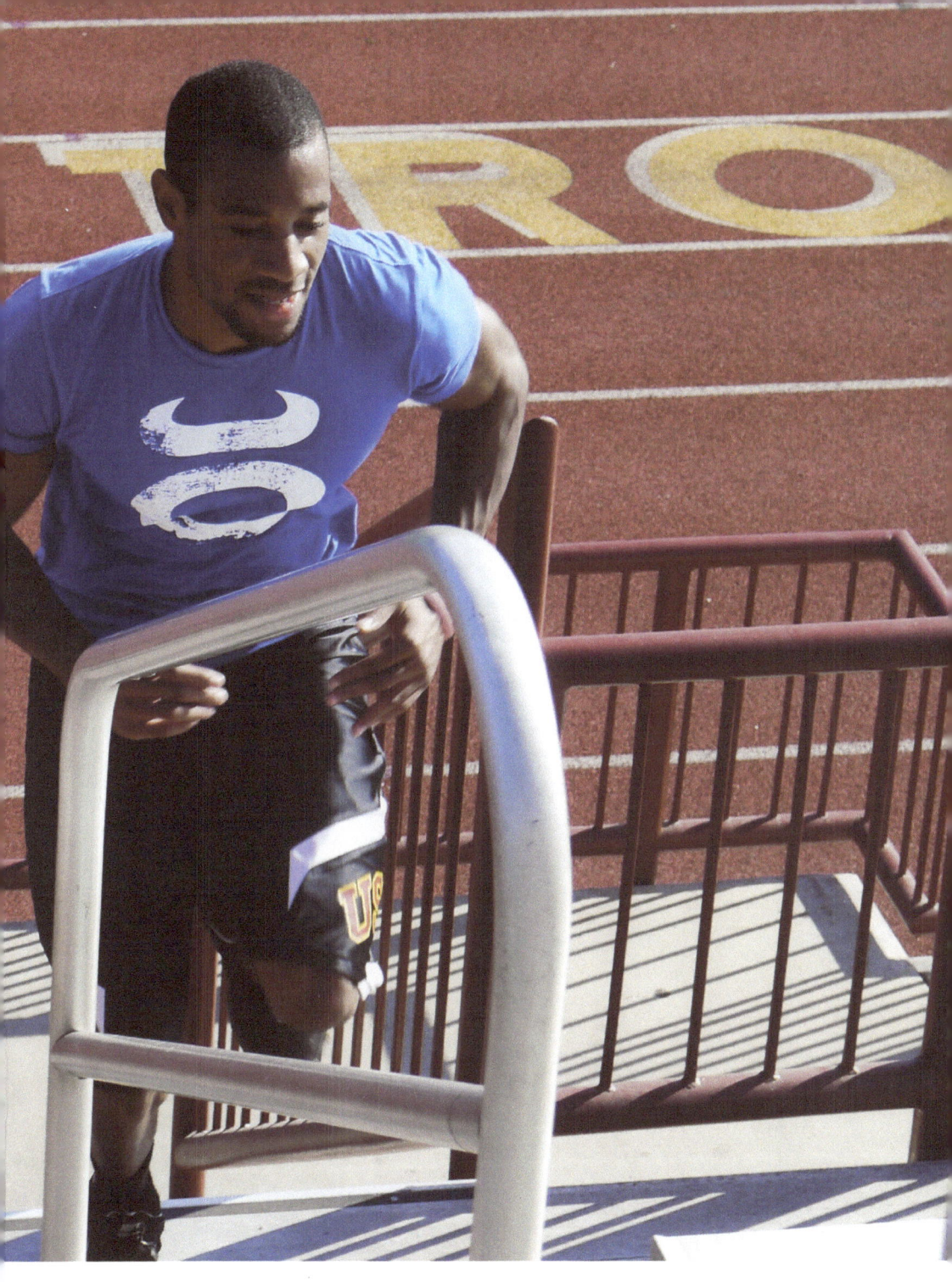

www.ingramcontent.com/pod-product-compliance
Lightning Source LLC
Chambersburg PA
CBHW040322010626
45792CB00024B/2097